BIONIC PETS

BY BETSY RATHBURN

BELLWETHER MEDIA · MINNEAPOLIS, MN

EPIC

EPIC

Action and adventure collide in EPIC. Plunge into a universe of powerful beasts, hair-raising tales, and high-speed excitement. Astonishing explorations await. Can you handle it?

This edition first published in 2021 by Bellwether Media, Inc.

Library of Congress Cataloging-in-Publication Data

Names: Rathburn, Betsy, author.
Title: Bionic pets / Betsy Rathburn.
Description: Minneapolis, MN : Bellwether Media, 2021. | Series: Epic.
   Cutting-edge technology | Includes bibliographical references and index.
   | Audience: Ages 7-12. | Audience: Grades 4-6. | Summary: "Engaging
   images accompany information about bionic pets. The combination of
   high-interest subject matter and light text is intended for students in
   grades 2 through 7"– Provided by publisher.
Identifiers: LCCN 2020001609 (print) | LCCN 2020001610 (ebook) | ISBN
   9781644872857 (library binding) | ISBN 9781681037486 (ebook)
Subjects: LCSH: Bionics–Juvenile literature. | Veterinary
   surgery–Juvenile literature. | Prosthesis–Juvenile literature. |
   Medical innovations–Juvenile literature.
Classification: LCC SF911 .R38 2021 (print) | LCC SF911 (ebook) | DDC
   636.089/7–dc23
LC record available at https://lccn.loc.gov/2020001609
LC ebook record available at https://lccn.loc.gov/2020001610

Editor: Kieran Downs   Designer: Josh Brink

Printed in the United States of America, North Mankato, MN.

TABLE OF CONTENTS

RACING AROUND

A dog chases a ball across a park. The dog is a blur as it races toward you. Watch out!
The dog's front legs are replaced by **prostheses**. These **limbs** help the dog go fast!

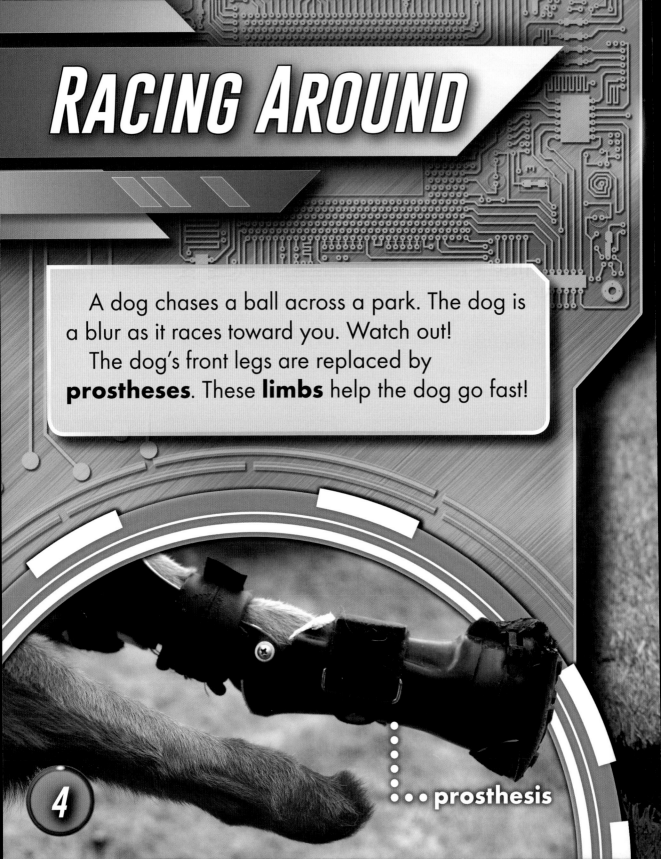

prosthesis

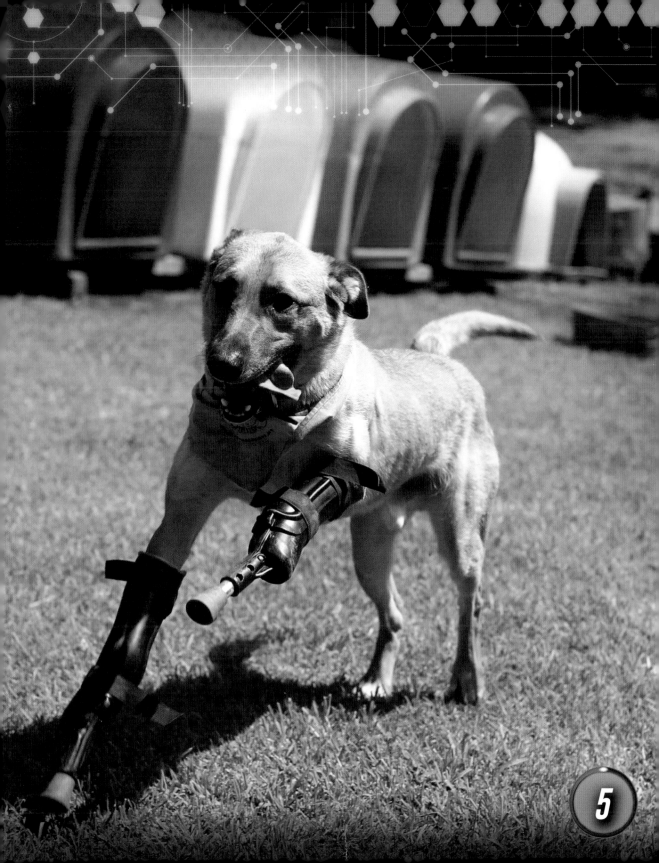

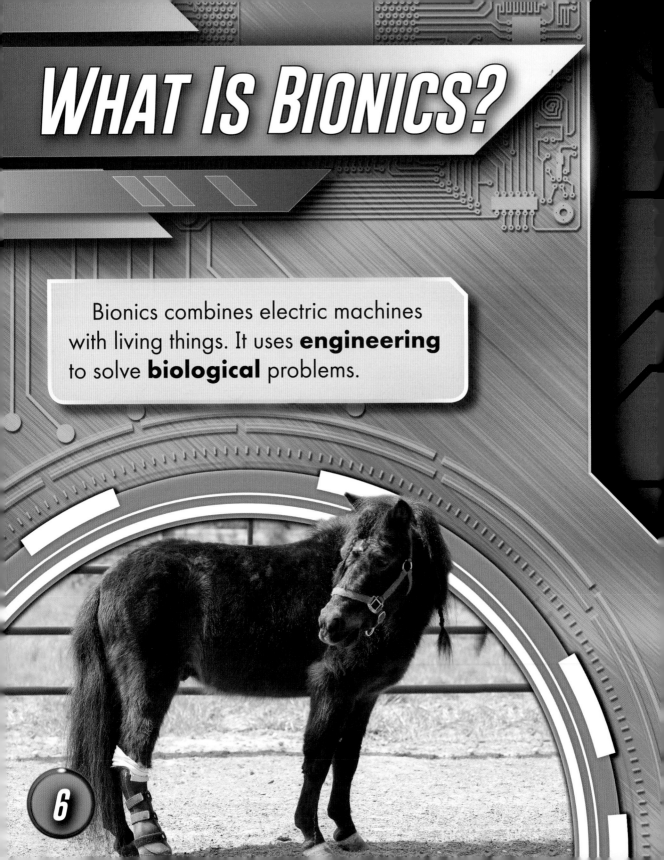

WHAT IS BIONICS?

Bionics combines electric machines with living things. It uses **engineering** to solve **biological** problems.

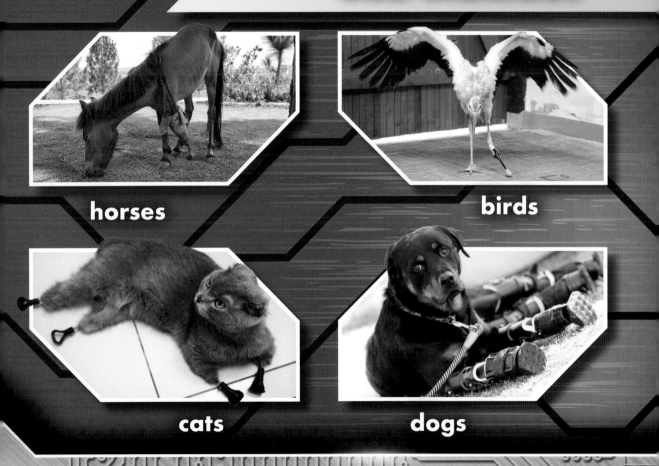

horses

birds

cats

dogs

Bionic machines work with prostheses. These help people and animals use their bodies.

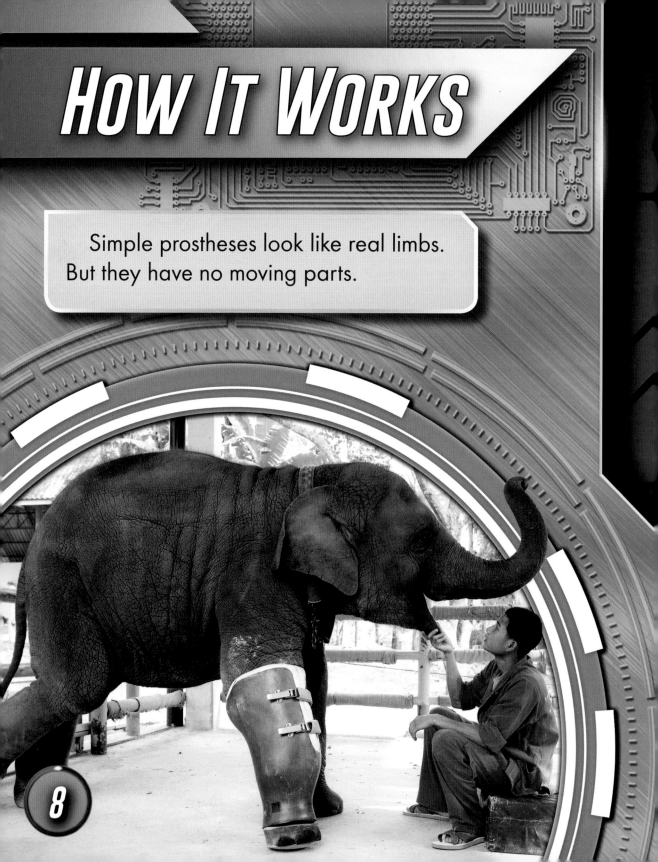

HOW IT WORKS

Simple prostheses look like real limbs. But they have no moving parts.

BODY-POWERED PROSTHESES

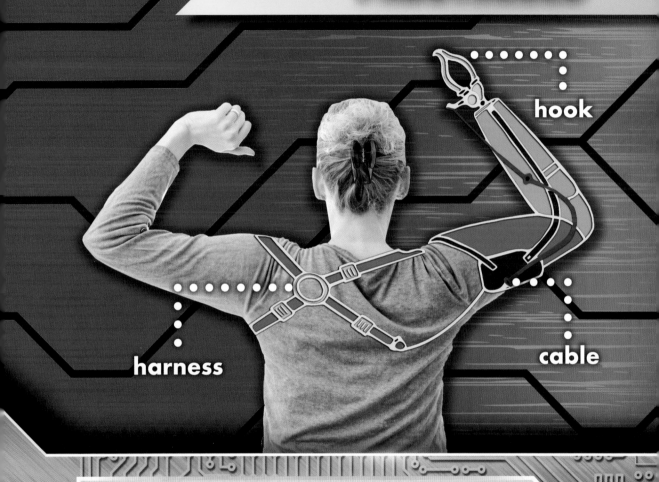

hook

harness

cable

Body-powered prostheses have moving parts. Users wear a **harness** to keep the prosthesis in place. Body movements move **cables** to move the prosthesis. Some prostheses have hooks to help grab!

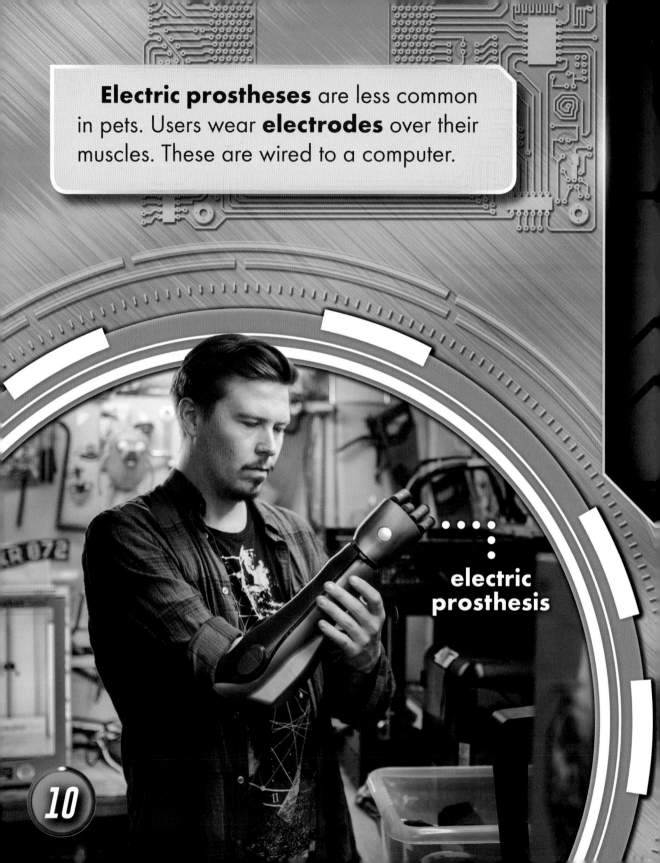

Electric prostheses are less common in pets. Users wear **electrodes** over their muscles. These are wired to a computer.

electric prosthesis

ELECTRIC PROSTHESES

electrode

wire

computer

Muscle movements send **signals** to the computer. The limb moves!

HISTORY

Prostheses have helped people for thousands of years. The first were made of wood and leather. But they did not have moving parts.

Advances came in the 1500s. A doctor created a **hinged** prosthetic hand. It could move!

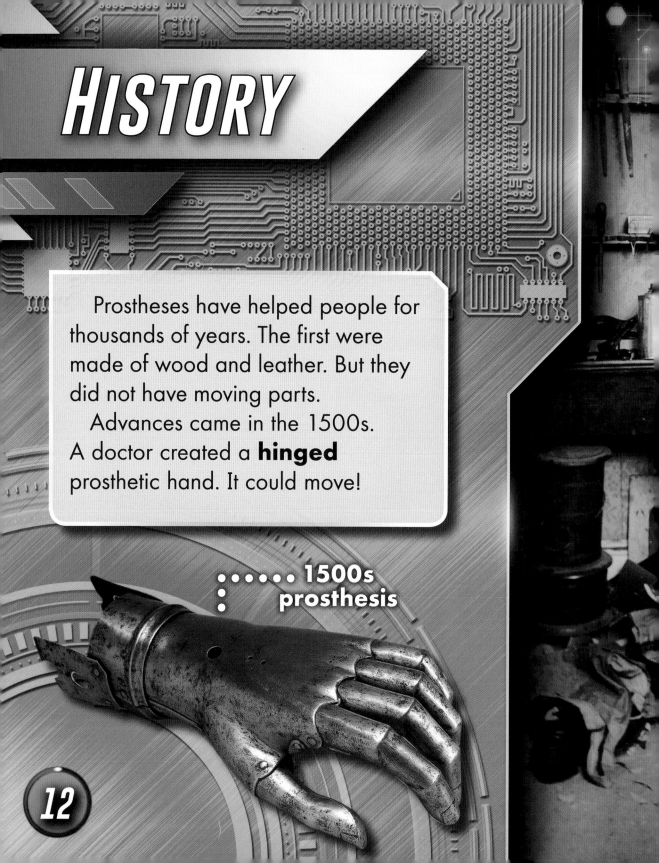

1500s prosthesis

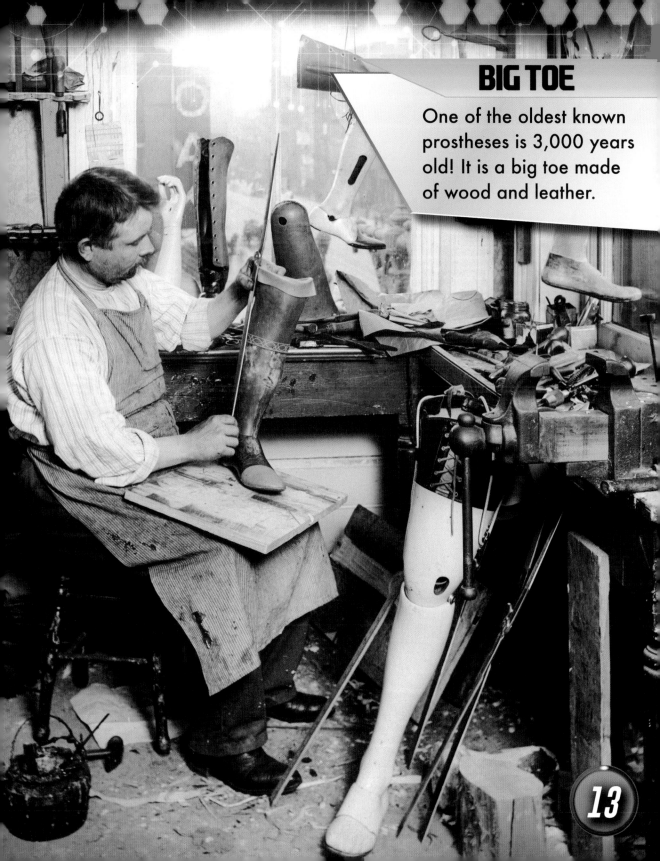

BIG TOE

One of the oldest known prostheses is 3,000 years old! It is a big toe made of wood and leather.

BIONICS TIMELINE

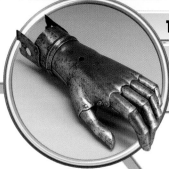

1500s
The first hinged prosthetic hand is used

2008
Beauty the eagle gets a prosthetic beak

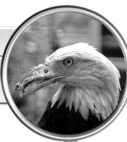

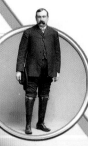

1800s
James Hanger creates a new prosthetic leg

2004
Fuji is first dolphin to get a prosthetic tail

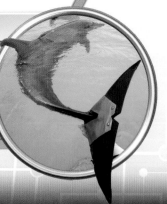

In the 1800s, James Hanger made a new prosthetic leg. Two hinges helped it move like a real leg.

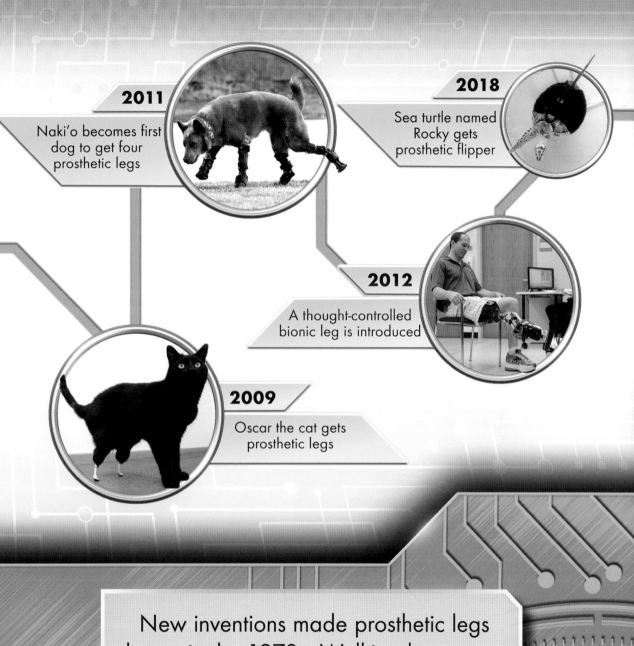

2011

Naki'o becomes first dog to get four prosthetic legs

2018

Sea turtle named Rocky gets prosthetic flipper

2012

A thought-controlled bionic leg is introduced

2009

Oscar the cat gets prosthetic legs

New inventions made prosthetic legs better in the 1970s. Walking became more comfortable!

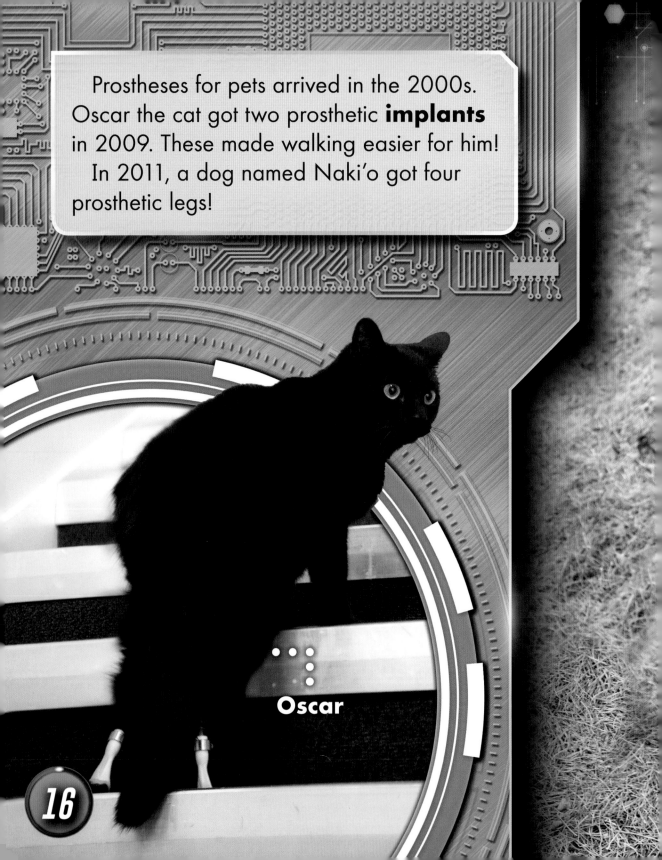

Prostheses for pets arrived in the 2000s. Oscar the cat got two prosthetic **implants** in 2009. These made walking easier for him! In 2011, a dog named Naki'o got four prosthetic legs!

Oscar

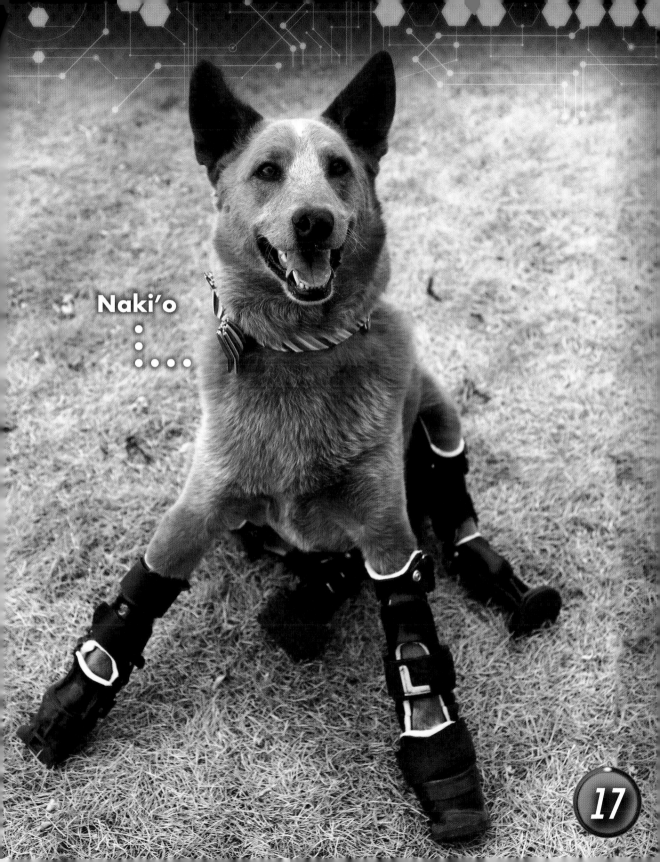

Naki'o

TECHNOLOGY OF TOMORROW

Technology continues to advance for people and pets. In 2012, scientists showed off a new bionic leg. The user moved the leg by thought!

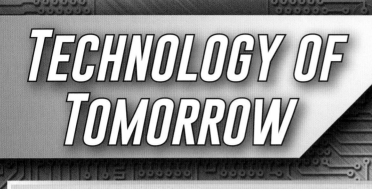

thought-controlled bionic leg

18

DOG ACTIVITIES

A study of 24 dogs found that most were able to do many activities after getting a prosthetic limb.

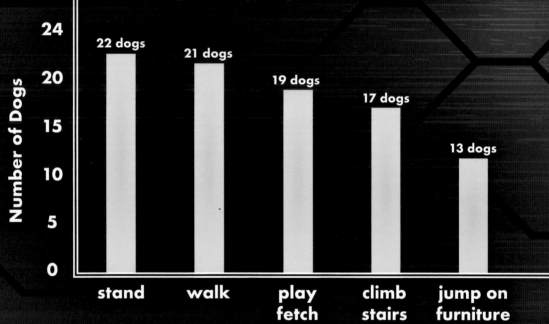

Number of Dogs

- 22 dogs — stand
- 21 dogs — walk
- 19 dogs — play fetch
- 17 dogs — climb stairs
- 13 dogs — jump on furniture

Many prostheses are now made by **3D printers**. This makes them cheaper. More pets can get new limbs!

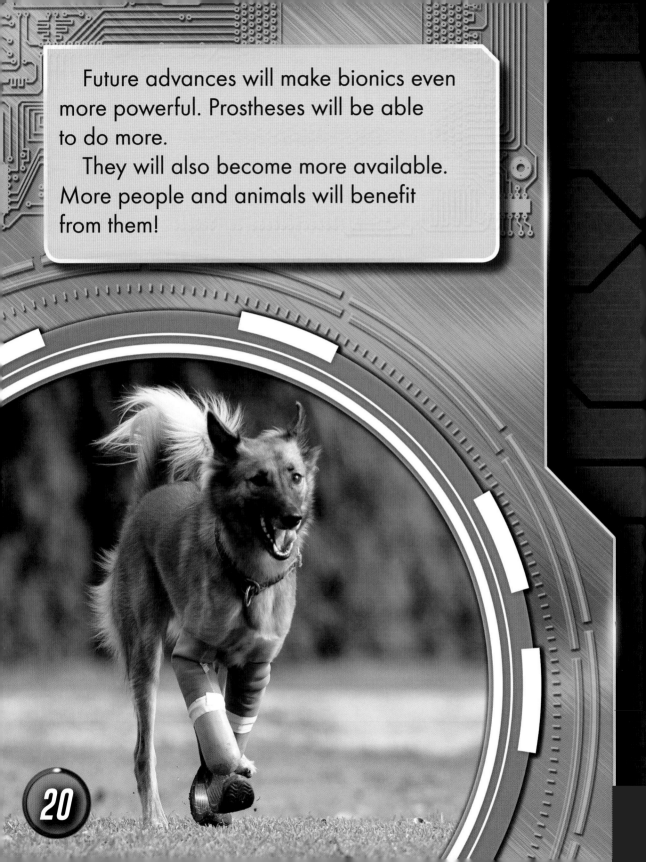

Future advances will make bionics even more powerful. Prostheses will be able to do more.

They will also become more available. More people and animals will benefit from them!

PROS AND CONS

Pros

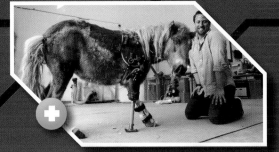

help people and
animals move

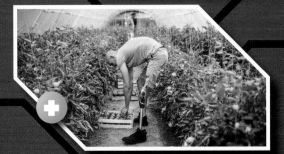

help people work

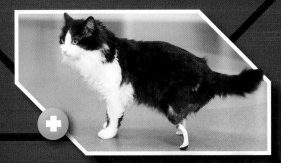

save injured
animals

Cons

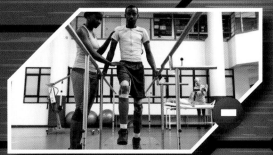

can be difficult
to use

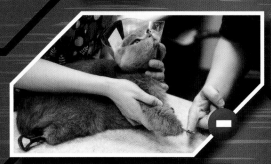

can be uncomfortable

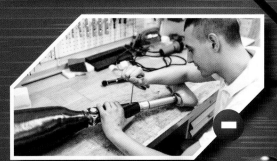

can need repair

GLOSSARY

3D printers—machines that use layers of plastic to create objects

biological—related to life and living things

body-powered prostheses—prostheses that are controlled by body movements

cables—strong wires or ropes

electric prostheses—prostheses that are controlled by electrical signals sent by body muscles to a computer on the prosthetic device

electrodes—objects through which electricity enters or leaves

engineering—the use of science and math to design and build things

harness—a device made to hold things to the body

hinged—connected to another object using a movable part called a hinge

implants—objects permanently inserted into the body

limbs—arms and legs

prostheses—human-made devices that replace or change missing or damaged body parts

signals—acts that tell someone or something what to do

To Learn More

AT THE LIBRARY

Bethea, Nikole Brooks. *Discover Bionics*. Minneapolis, Minn.: Lerner Publications, 2017.

Duhig, Holly. *Bionic Limbs*. New York, N.Y.: Gareth Stevens, 2018.

Furstinger, Nancy. *Unstoppable: True Stories of Amazing Bionic Animals*. Boston, Mass.: Houghton Mifflin Harcourt, 2017.

ON THE WEB

FACTSURFER

Factsurfer.com gives you a safe, fun way to find more information.

1. Go to www.factsurfer.com.

2. Enter "bionic pets" into the search box and click 🔍.

3. Select your book cover to see a list of related content.

23

INDEX

The images in this book are reproduced through the courtesy of: Lindsey Mladinich, cover; RICK WILKING, CIP, pp. 4, 15 (top left), 17; TOMAS BRAVO, p. 5; Fort Worth Star-Telegram, p. 6; Phatthanun Kaewsuwan, p. 7 (top left); picture alliance, p. 7 (top right); ITAR-TASS News Agency, p. 7 (bottom left); CB2/ZOB, pp. 7 (bottom right), 21 (left bottom); Barcroft, p. 8; AstroStar, p. 9; Red Bull, p. 10; PanicAttack, p. 11 (right); BigBlueStudio, p. 11 (left); Historical Views, p. 14 (top left); C. M. Bell Studio, p. 14 (bottom left); ISSEI KATO, p. 14 (bottom right); David Gowans, p. 14 (top right); Jim Incledon, p. 15 (bottom left); Brian Kersey, pp. 15 (top left), 18; Eric Gay, p. 15 (top right); rJP5\ZOB, p. 16; STRINGER, p. 20; KEVIN LAMARQUE, p. 21 (top left); wavebreakmedia, p. 21 (top right); South, p. 21 (middle left); TASS, p. 21 (middle right); hedgehog94, p. 21 (bottom right).